MW01242582

GOLO DIET

COOKBOOK FOR SENIORS

2 weeks meal plan with food list to Lose Weight and reduce the risk of chronic disease with GOLO friendly Recipes

Prof. AYDIN YENIL

TABLE OF CONTENTS

3

5

Chapter 1

INTRODUCTION

About the GOLO diet

The GOLO diet is a weight loss program that centers around controlling insulin levels to aid weight loss. Developed by a team of doctors, pharmacists, and nutritionists, the program aims to promote weight loss and enhance overall health.

The program includes a meal plan, supplements, and a support system to help users achieve their weight loss goals. The meal plan emphasizes whole foods, lean protein, healthy fats, and carbohydrates with a low glycemic index. The supplements are designed to support metabolism and regulate insulin.

According to its proponents, the GOLO diet is effective in helping people lose weight without requiring calorie counting or intense exercise. However, individual results may vary, as is the case with any weight loss program.

It's always advisable to consult with a healthcare provider before starting any new diet or weight loss program to ensure it is safe and suitable for your particular needs and health status.

Benefits of the GOLO diet for seniors

It's essential for seniors to consult with their healthcare provider before starting the GOLO diet, just like any other weight loss program or diet, to ensure that it is safe and suitable for their individual needs and health status

The GOLO diet may offer several potential advantages for seniors as it promotes a healthy and balanced approach to weight loss and nutrition.

• Improved Blood Sugar Control: By regulating insulin levels, the GOLO diet can be particularly beneficial for seniors who face a higher risk of developing insulin resistance and type 2 diabetes. This diet may help maintain stable blood sugar levels, thus reducing the risk of chronic health problems.

• Weight Loss: Being overweight can increase the likelihood of health issues such as heart disease, stroke, and joint problems, especially in seniors. The GOLO diet focuses on whole foods, lean protein, and low glycemic index carbohydrates, which may help seniors shed extra pounds.

• Enhanced Energy and Mood: Whole foods provide essential nutrients that promote energy levels and overall well-being, which can be especially valuable for seniors. Furthermore, the GOLO diet may help stabilize mood and reduce fatigue, factors that commonly affect seniors.

- Increased Social Support: The GOLO diet provides a support system that can benefit seniors by offering a community of like-minded individuals with similar health goals. This social support network enables seniors to share their experiences, offer encouragement, and find motivation to stick to their health and wellness goals.

Tips for following the GOLO diet as a senior

If you are a senior interested in following the GOLO diet,

Here are some tips to keep in mind:

- Consult with a healthcare provider: Before starting any new diet or weight loss program, it is crucial to speak with a healthcare provider to ensure that it is safe and appropriate for your individual needs and health status.

- Start slowly: The GOLO diet emphasizes a gradual and sustainable approach to weight loss. Seniors may find it helpful to start slowly and gradually incorporate the meal plan and supplements into their routine.

- Focus on whole foods: The GOLO diet emphasizes whole foods, lean protein, healthy fats, and low glycemic index carbohydrates. Seniors should aim to incorporate these foods into their meals as much as possible and limit processed foods and added sugars.

- Stay hydrated: Drinking enough water is essential for overall health and weight loss. Seniors should aim to drink at least 8-10 glasses of water per day and limit sugary beverages like soda and juice.

• Stay active: Regular physical activity is essential for weight loss and overall health. Seniors should aim to incorporate regular exercise into their routine, even if it's just a short walk or gentle yoga.

• Seek support: The GOLO diet offers a support system, including an online community, to help users stay motivated and on track. Seniors may find it helpful to connect with others who are also following the program and share their experiences and tips.

By following these tips, seniors can successfully adopt the GOLO diet and experience the potential benefits it offers for weight loss and overall health.

Chapter 2

GOLO-friendly Breakfast recipes

Spinach and Feta Omelet

Ingredients:

2 eggs

1 cup fresh spinach

1/4 cup crumbled feta cheese

1/4 tsp garlic powder

Salt and pepper to taste

1 tsp olive oil

Instructions:

- In a bowl, whisk together the eggs, garlic powder, salt, and pepper.
- Heat the olive oil in a nonstick pan over medium-high heat.

- Add the spinach and cook until wilted, about 2-3 minutes.
- Pour the egg mixture over the spinach and cook until the bottom is set, about 2-3 minutes.
- Flip the omelet and sprinkle the feta cheese on top.
- Cook until the cheese is melted and the egg is cooked through, about 2-3 minutes.
- Serve hot.

Nutritional Information:

Calories: 280 | Carbohydrates: 4g | Fat: 22g | Protein: 18g | Fiber: 1g | Sugar: 2g

Peanut Butter Banana Smoothie

Ingredients:

1 banana

1 tbsp peanut butter

1/2 cup unsweetened almond milk

1/4 cup plain Greek yogurt

1/2 tsp vanilla extract

1/2 tsp cinnamon

1 cup ice

Instructions:

- Blend all the ingredients together in a blender until smooth.
- Serve cold.

Nutritional Information:

Calories: 260 | Carbohydrates: 24g | Fat: 11g | Protein: 16g | Fiber: 4g | Sugar: 12g

Avocado and Egg Toast

Ingredients:

1 slice whole grain bread

1/2 avocado, mashed

1 egg

Salt and pepper to taste

1 tsp olive oil

Instructions:

- Toast the bread.
- In a nonstick pan, heat the olive oil over medium-high heat.
- Crack the egg into the pan and cook to your liking.
- Spread the mashed avocado on the toast.
- Place the cooked egg on top.
- Sprinkle with salt and pepper.
- Serve hot.

Nutritional Information:

Calories: 350 | Carbohydrates: 20g | Fat: 26g | Protein: 12g | Fiber: 8g | Sugar: 2g

Blueberry Overnight Oats

Ingredients:

1/2 cup rolled oats

1/2 cup unsweetened almond milk

1/4 cup plain Greek yogurt

1/2 cup fresh blueberries

1 tsp honey

Instructions:

- In a jar or container, mix together the oats, almond milk, and Greek yogurt.
- Stir in the blueberries and honey.
- Cover and refrigerate overnight.

- Serve cold.

Nutritional Information:

Calories: 260 | Carbohydrates: 38g | Fat: 6g | Protein: 12g | Fiber: 7g | Sugar: 14g

Tofu Scramble

Ingredients:

1/2 block firm tofu

1/4 cup chopped onion

1/4 cup chopped bell pepper

1/4 cup chopped mushrooms

1/4 tsp turmeric

Salt and pepper to taste

1 tsp olive oil

Instructions:

- In a nonstick pan, heat the olive oil
- Add the chopped onion, bell pepper, and mushrooms. Cook until the vegetables are tender, about 5-7 minutes.
- Crumble the tofu into the pan and sprinkle with turmeric, salt, and pepper. Stir well to combine.
- Cook for another 5-7 minutes or until the tofu is heated through.
- Serve hot.

Nutritional Information:

Calories: 170 | Carbohydrates: 8g | Fat: 11g | Protein: 12g | Fiber: 3g | Sugar: 3g

Chapter 3

GOLO-friendly Lunch recipes

Grilled Chicken and Vegetable Kabobs

Ingredients:

8 oz boneless, skinless chicken breast, cut into cubes

1/2 red onion, cut into cubes

1/2 bell pepper, cut into cubes

1/2 zucchini, sliced

1/2 tsp garlic powder

Salt and pepper to taste

1 tsp olive oil

Instructions:

- Preheat grill to medium-high heat.

- Thread the chicken, onion, bell pepper, and zucchini onto skewers.
- Brush with olive oil and sprinkle with garlic powder, salt, and pepper.
- Grill for 10-12 minutes, turning occasionally, or until the chicken is cooked through.
- Serve hot.

Nutritional Information:

Calories: 300 | Carbohydrates: 11g | Fat: 10g | Protein: 39g | Fiber: 3g | Sugar: 6g

Mediterranean Salad

Ingredients:

2 cups mixed greens

1/2 cup cherry tomatoes, halved

1/4 cup sliced cucumber

1/4 cup crumbled feta cheese

1/4 cup sliced Kalamata olives

2 tbsp olive oil

1 tbsp balsamic vinegar

Salt and pepper to taste

Instructions:

- In a large bowl, mix together the greens, tomatoes, cucumber, feta cheese, and olives.
- In a small bowl, whisk together the olive oil, balsamic vinegar, salt, and pepper.
- Drizzle the dressing over the salad and toss to combine.
- Serve cold.

Nutritional Information:

Calories: 260 | Carbohydrates: 10g | Fat: 21g | Protein: 7g | Fiber: 3g | Sugar: 5g

Turkey Wrap

Ingredients:

1 whole grain wrap

2 oz turkey breast

1/4 cup sliced avocado

1/4 cup sliced cucumber

1/4 cup mixed greens

1 tbsp hummus

Instructions:

- Lay the wrap on a flat surface.
- Spread the hummus over the wrap.
- Layer the turkey, avocado, cucumber, and mixed greens on top.
- Roll the wrap tightly.
- Serve cold.

Nutritional Information:

Calories: 330 | Carbohydrates: 24g | Fat: 16g | Protein: 23g | Fiber: 10g | Sugar: 2g

Quinoa and Black Bean Salad

Ingredients:

1 cup cooked quinoa

1/2 cup canned black beans, rinsed and drained

1/2 cup chopped bell pepper

1/2 cup chopped cucumber

1/4 cup chopped red onion

1/4 cup chopped fresh cilantro

1 tbsp olive oil

1 tbsp lime juice

Salt and pepper to taste

Instructions:

- In a large bowl, mix together the quinoa, black beans, bell pepper, cucumber, red onion, and cilantro.
- In a small bowl, whisk together the olive oil, lime juice, salt, and pepper.
- Drizzle the dressing over the salad and toss to combine.
- Serve cold.

Nutritional Information:

Calories: 280 | Carbohydrates: 40g | Fat: 9g | Protein: 11g | Fiber: 11g | Sugar: 3g

Egg Salad Lettuce Wraps

Ingredients:

3 hard-boiled eggs, peeled and chopped

1/4 cup chopped celery

1 tbsp chopped chives

1 tbsp Dijon mustard

2 tbsp plain Greek yogurt

Salt and pepper to taste

4 large lettuce leaves

Instructions:

- In a medium bowl, mix together the eggs, celery, chives, Dijon mustard, Greek yogurt, salt, and pepper.
- Spoon the egg salad onto the lettuce leaves.
- Roll up the lettuce leaves.
- Serve cold.

Nutritional Information:

Calories: 200 | Carbohydrates: 5g | Fat: 12g | Protein: 15g | Fiber: 1g | Sugar: 2g

Chapter 4

Dinner recipes

Baked Salmon with Roasted Vegetables

Ingredients:

4 oz salmon fillet

1/2 cup cherry tomatoes

1/2 cup sliced zucchini

1/2 cup sliced bell pepper

1/4 cup chopped red onion

1 tbsp olive oil

Salt and pepper to taste

Instructions:

- Preheat oven to 400°F (200°C).

- In a baking dish, arrange the salmon fillet and vegetables.
- Drizzle with olive oil and sprinkle with salt and pepper.
- Bake for 20-25 minutes or until the salmon is cooked through.
- Serve hot.

Nutritional Information:

Calories: 300 | Carbohydrates: 12g | Fat: 18g | Protein: 22g | Fiber: 3g | Sugar: 6g

Grilled Chicken Caesar Salad

Ingredients:

4 oz boneless, skinless chicken breast

2 cups chopped romaine lettuce

1/4 cup shaved parmesan cheese

2 tbsp Caesar dressing

Salt and pepper to taste

Instructions:

- Preheat grill to medium-high heat.
- Season the chicken breast with salt and pepper.
- Grill for 6-8 minutes per side or until the chicken is cooked through.
- Let the chicken rest for 5 minutes, then slice into strips.
- In a large bowl, mix together the lettuce, parmesan cheese, and Caesar dressing.
- Add the sliced chicken and toss to combine.
- Serve cold.

Nutritional Information:

Calories: 300 | Carbohydrates: 6g | Fat: 17g | Protein: 30g | Fiber: 2g | Sugar: 2g

Turkey Chili

Ingredients:

1 lb ground turkey

1 can (14 oz) diced tomatoes

1 can (14 oz) kidney beans, rinsed and drained

1 can (14 oz) corn, drained

1/2 onion, chopped

2 garlic cloves, minced

2 tbsp chili powder

1 tsp cumin

Salt and pepper to taste

Instructions:

- In a large pot, cook the ground turkey over medium-high heat until browned.
- Add the onion and garlic and cook until the onion is softened.
- Add the diced tomatoes (with juice), kidney beans, corn, chili powder, cumin, salt, and pepper.
- Bring to a boil, then reduce heat and simmer for 15-20 minutes.
- Serve hot.

Nutritional Information:

Calories: 350 | Carbohydrates: 29g | Fat: 11g | Protein: 34g | Fiber: 8g | Sugar: 6g

Grilled Pork Tenderloin with Steamed Broccoli

Ingredients:

4 oz pork tenderloin

1 cup broccoli florets

1 tbsp olive oil

Salt and pepper to taste

Instructions:

- Preheat grill to medium-high heat.
- Rub the pork tenderloin with olive oil and sprinkle with salt and pepper.
- Grill for 15-20 minutes, turning occasionally, or until the pork is cooked through.
- In a steamer basket, steam the broccoli for 5-7 minutes or until tender.
- Serve hot.

Nutritional Information:

Calories: 300 | Carbohydrates: 6g | Fat: 14g | Protein: 35

Quinoa Stuffed Bell Peppers

Ingredients:

2 bell peppers, halved and seeded

1/2 cup quinoa

1 cup vegetable broth

1/2 onion, chopped

1 garlic clove, minced

1/2 cup chopped spinach

1/2 cup diced tomatoes

1/4 cup crumbled feta cheese

Salt and pepper to taste

Instructions:

- Preheat oven to 375°F (190°C).
- In a small saucepan, bring the quinoa and vegetable broth to a boil.

32

- Reduce heat and simmer for 15-20 minutes or until the quinoa is cooked through.
- In a skillet, sauté the onion and garlic until the onion is softened.
- Add the spinach and diced tomatoes and cook until the spinach is wilted.
- Add the cooked quinoa to the skillet and stir to combine.
- Spoon the quinoa mixture into the bell pepper halves.
- Sprinkle with feta cheese and salt and pepper.
- Bake for 20-25 minutes or until the bell peppers are tender.
- Serve hot.

Nutritional Information:

Calories: 250 | Carbohydrates: 30g | Fat: 8g | Protein: 12g | Fiber: 6g | Sugar: 7g

Chapter 5

GOLO-friendly Snack recipes

Apple and Peanut Butter

Ingredients:

1 medium apple, sliced

1 tbsp natural peanut butter

Instructions:

- Spread peanut butter on apple slices.
- Enjoy as a snack.

Nutritional Information:

Calories: 180 | Carbohydrates: 21g | Fat: 9g | Protein: 4g | Fiber: 5g | Sugar: 14g

Greek Yogurt with Berries and Almonds

Ingredients:

1/2 cup plain Greek yogurt

1/2 cup mixed berries (blueberries, strawberries, raspberries)

1 tbsp sliced almonds

Instructions:

- Spoon Greek yogurt into a bowl.
- Top with mixed berries and sliced almonds.
- Enjoy as a snack.

Nutritional Information:

Calories: 150 | Carbohydrates: 15g | Fat: 6g | Protein: 11g | Fiber: 4g | Sugar: 7g

Hummus and Carrots

Ingredients:

2 tbsp hummus

1 cup baby carrots

Instructions:

- Dip baby carrots in hummus.
- Enjoy as a snack.

Nutritional Information:

Calories: 90 | Carbohydrates: 12g | Fat: 4g | Protein: 2g | Fiber: 4g | Sugar: 5g

Hard Boiled Eggs with Avocado

Ingredients:

2 hard boiled eggs

1/2 avocado, sliced

Instructions:

Slice hard boiled eggs in half.

Top with sliced avocado.

Enjoy as a snack.

Nutritional Information:

Calories: 210 | Carbohydrates: 8g | Fat: 17g | Protein: 9g | Fiber: 6g | Sugar: 1g

Cottage Cheese with Pineapple

Ingredients:

1/2 cup low-fat cottage cheese

1/2 cup diced pineapple

Instructions:

- Spoon cottage cheese into a bowl.
- Top with diced pineapple.
- Enjoy as a snack.

Nutritional Information:

Calories: 120 | Carbohydrates: 14g | Fat: 1g | Protein: 14g | Fiber: 1g | Sugar: 12g

Trail Mix

Ingredients:

1/4 cup unsalted almonds

1/4 cup unsalted cashews

1/4 cup unsalted pumpkin seeds

1/4 cup unsweetened dried cranberries

Instructions:

- Mix all ingredients in a bowl.
- Enjoy as a snack.

Nutritional Information:

Calories: 260 | Carbohydrates: 18g | Fat: 19g | Protein: 8g | Fiber: 3g | Sugar: 10g

Chapter 6

GOLO-friendly desserts

Chocolate Avocado Pudding

Ingredients:

1 ripe avocado

1/4 cup unsweetened cocoa powder

1/4 cup honey

1/4 cup almond milk

Instructions:

- Cut avocado in half and remove pit.
- Scoop out avocado flesh and add to blender.
- Add cocoa powder, honey, and almond milk to blender.
- Blend until smooth.

- Chill in refrigerator for at least 1 hour before serving.

Nutritional Information:

Calories: 290 | Carbohydrates: 40g | Fat: 15g | Protein: 5g | Fiber: 10g | Sugar: 27g

Baked Apples with Cinnamon

Ingredients:

2 medium apples

1 tsp cinnamon

1 tbsp honey

Instructions:

- Preheat oven to 350°F (175°C).
- Cut apples in half and remove core.
- Place apple halves in a baking dish.
- Sprinkle cinnamon and drizzle honey over apples.

- Bake for 25-30 minutes, or until apples are tender.

Nutritional Information:

Calories: 160 | Carbohydrates: 44g | Fat: 1g | Protein: 1g | Fiber: 7g | Sugar: 34g

Strawberry Chia Seed Pudding

Ingredients:

1 cup unsweetened almond milk

1/4 cup chia seeds

1/4 cup sliced strawberries

1 tsp honey

Instructions:

- Combine almond milk, chia seeds, and honey in a bowl.
- Stir well and let sit for 10 minutes.

- Stir in sliced strawberries.
- Chill in refrigerator for at least 1 hour before serving.

Nutritional Information:

Calories: 200 | Carbohydrates: 23g | Fat: 11g | Protein: 6g | Fiber: 11g | Sugar: 8g

Banana Oat Cookies

Ingredients:

2 ripe bananas, mashed

1 cup rolled oats

1/4 cup raisins

Instructions:

- Preheat oven to 350°F (175°C).
- Mix mashed bananas, rolled oats, and raisins in a bowl.

- Spoon mixture onto a baking sheet lined with parchment paper.
- Bake for 15-20 minutes, or until cookies are golden brown.

Nutritional Information:

Calories: 120 | Carbohydrates: 25g | Fat: 1g | Protein: 3g | Fiber: 3g | Sugar: 11g

Greek Yogurt and Berry Parfait

Ingredients:

1/2 cup plain Greek yogurt

1/2 cup mixed berries (blueberries, strawberries, raspberries)

1/4 cup granola

Instructions:

- Spoon Greek yogurt into a glass.
- Top with mixed berries and granola.

43

- Repeat layers until glass is full.

- Enjoy as a dessert.

Nutritional Information:

Calories: 230 | Carbohydrates: 35g | Fat: 4g | Protein: 14g | Fiber: 6g | Sugar: 14g

Chapter 7

2-week GOLO meal plan for seniors

This meal plan is just a sample and can be customized based on individual dietary needs and preferences. It is important for seniors to consult with their healthcare provider or a registered dietitian before starting any new diet or meal plan.

Week 1:

Monday:

Breakfast: Greek yogurt with berries and almonds

Lunch: Grilled chicken salad with mixed greens, cherry tomatoes, and balsamic vinaigrette

Dinner: Baked salmon with roasted asparagus and quinoa

Snack: Apple slices with almond butter

Dessert: Dark chocolate square

Tuesday:

Breakfast: Scrambled eggs with spinach and mushrooms

Lunch: Turkey wrap with hummus, avocado, and veggies

Dinner: Pork tenderloin with roasted Brussels sprouts and sweet potato

Snack: Cottage cheese with pineapple

Dessert: Fresh fruit salad

Wednesday:

Breakfast: Oatmeal with banana and walnuts

Lunch: Tuna salad with mixed greens and whole-grain crackers

Dinner: Beef stir-fry with broccoli, peppers, and brown rice

Snack: Carrots and hummus

Dessert: Greek yogurt with honey and cinnamon

Thursday:

Breakfast: Smoothie with spinach, berries, almond milk, and protein powder

Lunch: Grilled cheese sandwich with tomato soup

Dinner: Grilled shrimp skewers with mixed veggies and quinoa

Snack: Trail mix with nuts and dried fruit

Dessert: Frozen yogurt with berries

Friday:

Breakfast: Cottage cheese with peach slices and granola

Lunch: Chicken Caesar salad with whole-grain croutons

Dinner: Baked chicken with roasted root vegetables and brown rice

Snack: Edamame

Dessert: Banana with almond butter and honey

Saturday:

Breakfast: Veggie omelet with whole-grain toast

Lunch: Quinoa salad with chickpeas, cucumber, and feta cheese

Dinner: Beef chili with mixed veggies and brown rice

Snack: Hard-boiled egg

Dessert: Baked apple with cinnamon

Sunday:

Breakfast: Greek yogurt with granola and fresh berries

Lunch: Grilled chicken wrap with mixed greens and avocado

Dinner: Grilled steak with roasted veggies and sweet potato

Snack: Sliced cucumbers with tzatziki sauce

Dessert: Dark chocolate covered strawberries

Week 2:

Monday:

Breakfast: Smoothie with banana, peanut butter, and protein powder

Lunch: Turkey and cheese sandwich with veggies and hummus

Dinner: Baked cod with roasted Brussels sprouts and quinoa

Snack: Apple slices with cheese

Dessert: Fresh fruit salad

Tuesday:

Breakfast: Scrambled eggs with spinach and tomatoes

Lunch: Quinoa and black bean salad with avocado and salsa

Dinner: Chicken stir-fry with mixed veggies and brown rice

Snack: Greek yogurt with granola and berries

Dessert: Frozen yogurt with fruit

Wednesday:

Breakfast: Oatmeal with berries and almond butter

Lunch: Tuna salad with mixed greens and whole-grain crackers

Dinner: Beef and broccoli stir-fry with brown rice

Snack: Carrots and hummus

Dessert: Baked apple with cinnamon and honey

Thursday:

Breakfast: Smoothie with spinach, berries, almond milk, and protein powder

Lunch: Grilled cheese sandwich with tomato soup

Dinner: Grilled shrimp skewers with mixed veggies and quinoa

Snack: Trail mix with nuts and dried fruit

Dessert: Fresh fruit salad

Friday:

Breakfast: Cottage cheese with peach slices and granola

Lunch: Chicken Caesar salad with whole-grain croutons

Dinner: Baked salmon with roasted root vegetables and quinoa

Snack: Edamame

Dessert: Greek yogurt with honey and cinnamon

Saturday:

Breakfast: Veggie omelet with whole-grain toast

Lunch: Lentil soup with whole-grain crackers

Dinner: Grilled chicken with roasted veggies and sweet potato

Snack: Sliced cucumbers with tzatziki sauce

Dessert: Dark chocolate covered strawberries

Sunday:

Breakfast: Greek yogurt with granola and fresh berries

Lunch: Turkey and cheese wrap with veggies and hummus

Dinner: Beef stew with mixed veggies and brown rice

Snack: Hard-boiled egg

Dessert: Fresh fruit salad

Chapter 8

Conclusion

To summarize, the Golo diet cookbook for seniors is an excellent dietary option for older adults seeking to enhance their health and sustain a healthy weight. The program emphasizes balanced meals that are nutrient-rich and low in processed foods, sugar, and unhealthy fats.

With a variety of delicious, easy-to-prepare recipes, this Golo diet cookbook is tailored to seniors' unique nutritional requirements.

Additionally, the Golo diet program provides seniors with practical recommendations and guidance to adopt healthy lifestyle habits that complement the diet and enhance health outcomes.

While the Golo diet may not be suitable for all individuals, particularly those with specific dietary restrictions or medical concerns, it is generally a safe and effective dietary option for seniors looking to improve their health and well-being. However, it is advisable to seek advice from a healthcare provider before embarking on any new dietary or exercise regimen.

In conclusion, the Golo diet cookbook for seniors is a valuable resource for older adults seeking to lead a healthy lifestyle and maintain their quality of life. By adhering to the principles of the program and integrating the recommended lifestyle habits, seniors can achieve optimal health and well-being during their golden years.

Made in the USA
Middletown, DE
06 November 2023